7 SECRETS
DOCTORS DON'T WANT
YOU TO KNOW
ABOUT LOSING WEIGHT
PERMANENTLY

DR. KATHLEEN NASH, D.C.

7 SECRETS DOCTORS DON'T WANT YOU TO KNOW ABOUT LOSING WEIGHT PERMANENTLY

PacChiropractic LLC
Dr. Kathleen Nash, D.C.
204 W. Pacific Ave
Henderson, NV 89015
(866) 515-0101

HEALTH & FITNESS / Diet & Nutrition / Weight Loss: the best way to lose weight and keep it off / Dr. Kathleen Nash, D.C. -1st. ed.

ISBN-13: 978-1530710119
ISBN-10: 1530710111

Printed in the United States of America

CONTENTS

FOREWARD

It is my mission to free our country from the bonds of obesity in all its forms. And to stop the "lose weight / gain weight" cycle so people can lead healthy, productive lives. The truth is there is no easy solution to our obesity epidemic. While this book gives information that i think is left out of many weight loss programs, addressing specific metabolic conditions is outside the scope of this book and your specific metabolic issues should be addressed by a health care professional before starting any weight loss program.

DISCLAIMER

Please note that individual results when embarking on a health journey vary from person to person. Depending on personal medical history or specific health conditions, some people need strategic medical intervention, including medication and in extreme cases, surgery. This book is in no way intended as medical advise therefore please do not discontinue or change dosages of all prescribed medication without seeking professional advise from someone who knows your health history. This book can in no way substitute for competent medical treatment.

WARNING

Dietary changes and nutritional supplementation can be extremely effective in changing the symptomatology of Metabolic Syndrome including: losing body fat, blood sugar levels, blood pressure, and cholesterol. Therefore if you are on specific medication a consultation with your physician to monitor medication dosages may be warranted. Avoiding this step could be extremely harmful and potentially lead to overdosing. Please make sure to consult with your health care professional.

Introduction

My name is Dr. Kathleen Nash and I'm a chiropractic physician. I have been in private practice since 2001, but since 2013 my specialty has been metabolic weight loss. This is because in 2009 I lost 80 pounds and went from a size 20 to a size 8 and did something I'd never been able to do before. I kept the weight off. You see, the national statistics in our country (depending on where you look, because they can vary.) say that 95% of people who lose weight in the United States gain it back within one year. Those are dismal results and, chances are if you're reading this book, you fall into that 95% category. So what did I go to finally lose it for good? I discovered the Seven Secrets. Once I applied them not only was I able to lose weight, but I did it without hunger, without cravings, no drugs, no surgery. But more on that later..

For now lets start at the beginning. I started gaining weight was I was 8 years old. This was at a time when most kids were not fat. Now it's everywhere, and not only are our children suffering from being overweight and obese, but also have metabolic conditions such as: type II diabetes, fatty liver, and a variety of cardiovascular and pulmonary problems. I was on my first diet when I was 9. It was your typical low calorie, do it yourself, created by my mom kind of diet. And it worked!

At least until I stop doing it. And then the weight came right back on. And from age 9 I started a pattern of yo-yo dieting, trying every diet you that came out, losing weight only to gain it back plus more. It culminated in me becoming a 230 pound doctor trying to convince my patients to do preventative care. Not a very good role model.

And with every new diet I started I would dredge up my enthusiasm, muster up all my willpower and tell myself, "This time I will do it for sure! No matter what, no excuses I'm going to get it done." And with the inevitable failure that I would always experience when I would gain the weight back would also come all of the horrible negative emotions: the guilt, the shame, the sadness, and the feeling of hopelessness that I would never be able to fix this problem.

This leads us up to 2009 where, instead of constantly blaming myself for my failure, I started objectively looking around at my environment. What I started to realize was that the majority of people in my country were now at least classified as overweight (with a BMI of 26 or more) and over 25% of the country (7 out of 10) were classified as obese (BMI over 30). Not only we're regular people suffering from obesity, but our celebrities, the wealthy, and the privileged were suffering as well. People that we would consider had a wealth of resources at their fingertips, were definitely active, structured, and organized, and possessed a greater capability then we do to reach their goal weight and keep it off. So why was everybody so darn fat? And why could so many of us not keep it off for more than a year?

What I identified is a large part of what makes of this book. That there are specific metabolic conditions that, if aren't addressed and corrected, guarantees failure in weight loss for the long-term. When I applied new methods of losing weight that addressed these conditions to myself, *that's* when I finally started seeing long term success in and maintaining my goal weight.

Of course because I was actively treating patients, they were noticing the transformation I was experiencing, and also noticing that I was keeping the weight off. Many of them started to ask me what I was doing and if there was a way that I could create a program for them as well. By offering to do this for my existing patients, I was able to see that these metabolic problems could be identified and corrected in people besides me. My patients started to experience accelerated weight loss, they also did not have hunger or cravings, they did little or any exercise, and they too were able to beat the national statistics. And as an added bonus they were getting off medication and correcting chronic symptoms and disease.

In doing this, I slowly began to realize that many of the things we have been told to do to get healthy and lose weight were **flat out wrong.** At that point it became my mission to help as many people as I could overcome their specific issues that was preventing them from being not only as healthy as they wanted to be but to finally look and feel the way they wanted. It has been a liberating and rewarding experience, and a passion that I will probably pursue for the rest of my life.

This book is for anyone who has struggled with losing weight and keeping it off. It is for the person who is suffering from Metabolic Syndrome and it's associated symptoms: Weight gain, obesity, insulin resistance, type II diabetes, high blood pressure, high cholesterol, high triglycerides, heart disease, stroke, depressed immune function, depressed thyroid function, and even certain forms of cancer. It is for the person who is sick and tired of being sick and tired, who wants to transform their body and their health to levels they never thought possible.

Let's get started…

Chapter One

Are There Actually Factors Causing Me to Be Fat?

The bottom line is: Yes.

In my experience, I have identified that there are five different metabolic factors. These five metabolic factors that have an impact on our ability not only to lose weight, but to keep it off long-term, and three are absolutely critical. I'm going to get into those three in really big detail later on.

But the bottom line or the take-home message is this: if we're trying to lose weight and our ultimate goal is to keep it off, then these metabolic factors must be corrected. Otherwise, any weight that you do lose is either going to be slow, it's going to plateau often, and in 95 percent of the cases, will only be temporary, lasting less than a year.

Factor 1: Hormonal Imbalance

So lets start by identifying what "metabolic" means. Metabolism is the chemical processes that occur within a living body in order to maintain life, and a metabolic factor is an underlying circumstance, fact, or influence that contributes to how well the metabolism operates. The top three metabolic factors that I discuss here that are making people fat are: dietary hormones or hormonal imbalances, gross corporeal toxicity but especially in the fat cells and liver, and then the third one is the hypothalamic set point, which basically means that the hypothalamus uses a set-point to regulate the body's systems, including electrolyte and fluid balance, body temperature, blood pressure, and for the importance of our discussion here: body weight.

When I usually talk with a client about a metabolic program or metabolic issues I will get an argument from most that their problem is just a calories in / calories out issue. But remember, I played that game since I was 8 years old. The calories in, calories out method actually has a multitude of factors built into it that are both misleading and false.

So why would so many diet programs, including drastic forms of intervention such as bariatric surgery, continue to cling to this method as the gold standard?

Not wanting to sound like a conspiracy theorist, it really is a benefit to many different industries to put the blame on the dieter for the reason that they're heavy. We're constantly told our weight problems are because due to an overconsumption or an underutilization issue, meaning "I eat too much and I move too little."

But the bottom line is, the body is not a simple mathematical equation, and if calories in, calories out worked, then all of us would only have to diet one time, reach our goal weight, and we would stay there. But the truth of the matter is, it's an actually far more complicated process than just calories in, calories out. Which is why 95% of us fail when we employ this method. But the hidden benefit to calories in / calories out, for the diet industry anyway, is that they can continue to blame the dieter and have the dieter continually feel like a failure and come back and repeat the programs.

Now let's take a look at hormone imbalance. There are actually up to eight different hormones that can cause your body not only to suffer and not be able to lose weight, but not be able to keep it off, as well.

Three of them that we've identified — HGH, DHEA, and our sex hormones, whether it's testosterone for a male, or progesterone for a female — these are hormones that just naturally start depleting at 30 years of age. It's one of those things where we really don't have much control, and by the time we're 50, they reduce to half. This means to some degree, they are out of our control unless we supplement them externally, whether it's a cream, injection, or oral medication. Five other ones, however, are dietary related. So insulin, glucagon, leptin, ghrelin, and cortisol are the five dietary hormones, which is good news for us because it means that if we structure our diet a specific way, **we can have a direct impact** on the dietary hormones.

By the food intake, by the structure of the food that you're eating, by the timing of the food that you're eating, you can regulate and control these hormones, and what most of us don't realize is what a huge impact it has on not only how fast or slow we lose weight, but what type of weight are we losing.

Are we losing body fat? Are we losing muscle? Are we losing a mixture of both? If we're losing a mixture of both, what's the percentage? And so it's very important to recognize that, in terms of hormonal imbalance, the biggest one that drives all this dysfunction is insulin.

To keep it simple, insulin is a fat storage hormone, and glucagon is a fat burning hormone, and whenever you eat foods that trigger insulin to be in the bloodstream and stay there, your body has a very difficult time burning fat for fuel. This is because it's an inverse relationship. When insulin is present, glucagon has to be absent. It doesn't exist otherwise.

So one problem, a huge problem that we have in our country is that, for the most part, based on how we eat pretty much since the 1980's, our insulin levels remain high. The problem with insulin levels remaining high, it being a fat storage hormone, is it's going to suppress glucagon, the fat burning hormone.

Another problem is insulin interferes with a hormone called "leptin," which we didn't even know about until 1994. It comes directly out of our fat tissue and tells the brain how much fat we have in storage.

The problem with leptin is, when insulin is circulating in the bloodstream, not only does it encourage the body to store sugar (usually as body fat unless we're fairly active on a daily basis), but insulin also goes into the brain and blocks the receptor sites that leptin attaches to. As a result, the leptin signal telling us to stop eating and to stop storing more fat **cannot be heard.** This leads us to keep over eating and to keep storing more and more body fat.

The take home message here is when you eat foods that trigger an insulin response a cascade of nasty things happen in terms of losing or gaining body fat: you burn sugar instead of fat, your body takes extra energy and converts it to body fat and won't burn it, and when you're doing this on a meal-per-meal basis or a daily basis, you're also continuously blocking the brain's ability to recognize when you're full so you'll pretty much over eat every time you have a meal.

The last two hormones discussed here are ghrelin and cortisol. Cortisol is a stress hormone, so when we're under high periods of stress or continued high periods of stress, the cortisol hormone will actually cause us to deposit fat around the abdomen or belly. This causes an increased risk of cardiovascular disease, as well as a host of other problems outside of the scope of this book.

And then, ghrelin is a hormone produced by the stomach. Often called the 'hunger hormone' because it stimulates appetite, increases food intake, and promotes fat storage.

Factor 2: Toxicity

Toxicity is the 2nd major factor. The problem with toxicity is our bodies were really never designed to handle as much toxin as they do in our urban environment.

So if I'm talking to a female, for example, not only is she dealing with the urban environment that she's in and the toxins that are in our housing, our building materials, the pollutants in the air, and the chemicals and the insecticides in the food, I'm also dealing with somebody who probably introduces personalized toxins into her system.

For example, many women use dyes or bleaches on their hair. She probably wears cosmetics, puts on sunscreen, uses perfume and fragrances in her clothing and detergents, and things of that nature. And the problem with these materials is that they seep into the pores of the skin.

So as the body become bombarded with toxicity, it has to do something with that. We have several mechanisms designed to purge toxin from the body. The skin is one example, such as when we sweat. And another major player to remove toxin is the liver. Now, if the liver is overloaded with too much toxin, it's going to have two negative things happen to it, in terms of losing weight and keeping it off.

One, the body's going to start depositing the toxin into the fat cells directly. Mainly because fat cells are inert, meaning they don't do much, so the body puts the toxin in there because it basically is safeguarded from it. If toxin is allowed to circulate throughout the body, it's going to cause a problem basically the body thinks, "I have to put this somewhere so I don't get sick so I'm going to put it in a relatively low-active tissue. Ah, here's some fat. I'll put it here."

The second problem, which is huge, is that the toxin begins to back up in the liver. The liver is the only organ that can break down and metabolize body fat, so if your liver cannot convert that body fat to fuel at a decent pace, it just gets reabsorbed back into the fat cells. So excessive toxicity will make the body resistant to releasing fat from the cells and the liver will be inefficient at breaking down and converting body fat to a fuel we can use. This results in being a deadly combination for anyone who wants to lose weight.

Factor 3: Set Point

Factor three is the body's set point. The body weight set point theory states that the body uses hormones, hunger, behavior changes and other physiologic mechanisms to "defend" a certain range of body weight and the percentage of body fat that we carry. In terms of physiologic mechanisms, there are actually three different parts of the brain that controls weight range and body fat percentage: the hypothalamus, which controls the pituitary gland, and then the pituitary gland that controls the thyroid gland.

What we've identified with the hypothalamus is that the longer you sit at any weight...it doesn't matter if you're at ideal weight, 100 pounds, 200 pounds, 500 pounds.

The longer you sit at any weight, the more you reprogram the hypothalamus that this is the weight that it is supposed to be at, and once that happens, the physiologic mechanisms that control metabolism: energy expenditure, hunger signals, hormone levels, etc. will adjusted to maintain that weight.

So the downside is, what we've often been told in the diet industry is that you can't change your set point. If a person hears that they have a set point, that they have no control over where their weight or body fat percentage is, then they just begin to accept that, "I'm destined to be fat, I will always be fat, and there's really no point for me to try and change anything if I'm going to just remain the same." Which really bothers me, because the diet industry and health industry like to give the impression that it can't be altered, that your body just has this natural set point, that it wants to stay a certain weight. This can can true because you don't know how to change it, the good news for people who want to get to a lower body fat range or a lower size is that it can be controlled, but it has to be controlled by a long-term management strategy.

Chapter Two

What Healthy Foods Are Secretly Causing Weight Gain?

Modified, Low-Fat Foods Are Causing Weight Gain

In the early 1980s, the government started to have more control and input in our diet and food supply. This was primarily based on the results of a study by a scientist named Ancel Keys called the "Seven Countries Study". In the study, it was determined that excessive fat, and especially saturated fat, in the diet was a direct contributor to obesity and, in particular, heart disease.

Shortly afterward, our processed food supply was completely overhauled as food manufacturers scrambled to remove the fat from our grocery store shelves. Since that time, not only have our processed foods been plagued with the words "low-fat," "fat-free," "lite," in an attempt for us to control our battle of the bulge, but obesity rates, heart disease, Type 2 Diabetes, and childhood obesity rates have also skyrocketed. Clearly something in the research was wrong.

Statistics also show that at the same time these low-fat or these modified low-fat foods have been introduced into our food supply, that our obesity didn't drop as we expected them to. Instead, the rates have climbed.

And this is because when the fat is deliberately taken out of a food, a lot of times the good texture and the flavor that accompanied it is also removed. The food ends up tasting flavorless, bland, and practically inedible. The food manufacturers know this.

So if a food manufacturer wants to sell a product that used to be high in fat and used to taste good, and now they have to create a lower-fat version, what they will do is replace the fat with sugar. And the problem is, when you put sugar into a food and when that sugar enters the body, it is quickly converted into fat, usually within 20 minutes, and it's the main reason that we see the obesity rates rising. So low-fat foods are actually a devil in disguise.

Artificial Sweeteners Can Make Me Fat

They absolutely can, and here's why.

First of all, what's an artificial sweetener? An artificial sweetener can be anything from saccharine, it can be Splenda, it can be aspartame, it can be Truvia, or Stevia. And the problem with the artificial sweeteners that we don't know — while they are zero-calorie or ultra-low calorie, like one calorie in an ounce or something like that — it's the sweet response that the brain has once we eat it.

When we take the artificial sweetener in, it might have zero calories, but the brain recognizes the taste of sweet, and the brain is smart and understands that, "If I taste sweet, that must mean calories are coming in, and because it's a sweet calorie, I need to secrete insulin."

But remember, we said insulin's our fat storage hormone.

Going for an example, let's say somebody drinks a diet Coke. It doesn't have any calories, but because it tasted sweet, the body secreted insulin, and now for the next few hours your

16

body's going to be storing fat because it tasted something sweet even though it was zero-calorie.

Is Sugar Really a Problem, or Not?

Sugar is a definite problem. It's the major contributor to obesity, not only in our country, but all over the world now, especially developing nations or countries that are more socioeconomically distressed. There are multiple reasons why sugar causes obesity. The first one I'll discuss is the body's biochemical response to sugar when it's eaten.

When the body eats refined sugar or sugar of any kind only the liver can process or metabolize it. However, sugar, refined carbohydrates, or sugar that has been stripped of fiber overloads the liver when it gets broken down, which is essentially in a nanosecond of entering the digestive system. As the liver gets overloaded, it has no choice but to incorporate insulin from the pancreas to help it control the massive rate that sugar is entering the bloodstream. The insulin's going to take that sugar and it's going to look to do three things with it.

1. "Can I burn it right away?"

For most of our population, the answer here is "no". If you're overweight, chances are you're sedentary to some degree and you can't burn the sugar off right away because you are not or have not been active enough to do so.

2. "Can I store it in muscle?"

If the body doesn't have an immediate energy demand tt's going to look to see if it can package it and store it for later. Imagine a little suitcase of muscle sugar that goes directly into our muscles. That's called "glycogen." It's the second storage site for sugar.

3. "Where's the last place I can store it?"

However, since the only way the body can create a little suitcase of muscle sugar is if you've emptied that suitcase beforehand, people who don't exercise or are not active regularly have little room in the second option. This means all of those calories that you're eating gets converted and stored as body fat.

Is There a Difference Between Refined Sugar and Natural Sugar?

No. For our intents and purposes in the scope of this book they're exactly the same.

Grains Can Make Me Fat

Most of my clients are pretty savvy and they understand that sugar, and even artificial sweeteners are contributing to their weight problem. A few of them are also aware of the "fat isn't really the issue" debate as well. But grains?The idea that whole grains can cause not only a weight problem, but all the metabolic conditions associated with it. Yeah. That's usually news to them. When we talk about a grain, basically, most people think wheat. Whether that's the white or wheat variety doesn't really matter. And because gluten (the substance present in cereal grains, especially wheat) and gluten intolerance has been making big headlines in the public health sector, food manufacturers have latched on to another money making idea and suddenly 'gluten-free' everything is on practically every aisle of the supermarket. But what we're talking about doesn't have to be just wheat. It can be any kind of grain. So it can be wheat, it can be a corn flour, it can be a barley or a rye flour, it can be an oat flour. It's what happens when the grain starts to digest that is the problem.

Certain foods, while they enter the body as a grain and they have a completely different taste from sugar, chemically are broken down in the exact same way. It's what the body does with the grain chemically, once it comes inside, that determines what's going to happen and how it will affect your weight and your health. What it eventually gets broken down into controls what your body is going to do with it.

Grains, and especially refined grains, because they're also a carbohydrate, get broken down into a sugar, and so ultimately it's the same effect. You can have three different foods on your plate, let's they're all grains. They taste different, they look different, they aren't even sweet.. but they will all do the same thing once they pass the throat. Actually even sooner than that; once they enter your mouth enzyme begin breaking them down in the same manner.

One food could be something simple, like corn flakes. One could be a whole-wheat pasta and another one can be an ear of corn, and the problem is, the minute — in the mouth, they taste like three different things, none of them are sweet. But, the minute it passes the throat, chemically, the body sees it as sugar and will do that same process to all three, whether it tastes sweet or not, whether it's labeled as sugar or not. Once these foods enter the body, they're converted to sugar. And they have the same effect on your weight and metabolism that sugar has. Damaged, diseased, and fat.

Processed Diet Foods Keep Me Fat

The problem with the processed diet foods is the food manufacturers know that not only is this food supposed to cause you to lose weight, but you've got to be able to digest it and it's got to be palatable. So in order to do that, several things happen to the food. One, it's highly processed. The higher the processing content, the more quickly it's converted to energy, which means the more quickly it's converted to sugar and the quicker your body's going to convert it to body fat.

The second problem is they're all high in chemical agents, they're all high in preservatives, and these toxins come into the body and contribute to the toxicity level of the body.

So they clog up the liver, they cause even more toxins to be deposited into the liver, they cause even more toxins to be deposited into the fat cells, and any fat cell that has an accumulation of toxin, the body's going to be resistant to burning.

Processed foods are also designed to make you overeat. A food manufacturer, whether he's selling a diet food or a gourmet food has one overall goal in mind. To increase the profits for his company. Over the course of human history our bodies have evolved to regulate energy consumption and expenditure. However, modern science and food science techniques have created an exorbitant amount of "hyper-palatable" foods. These foods overstimulate the brain with a combination of sugar, salt, fat, and chemical additives that are formulated and field tested until they find the "bliss point". This is the maximum amount of the food you'll eat before your brain will tell you to stop eating. Designed to fatten up their bottom line... and yours.

Chapter Three

How Could Exercise Keep You Fat?

In order to talk about exercise and it's overall impact on the rate or ability for your body to lose weight, we first have to define what "exercise" is. So really, exercise is any activity requiring physical effort. Usually carried out to sustain or improve health and fitness. It's this effort that makes the body burn a calorie, which for the scope of this book is just a unit of energy.

Therefore, exercise doesn't necessarily mean that someone is in the gym, or playing sports, or weight training. It can be something as simple as…cleaning the houser a physical job. The amount of energy it's going to take, besides your basic metabolic function, any voluntary active muscle contraction can be defined as an exercise.

So that being said, let's talk about the types of exercise. Mainly, we usually break it up into two big categories. One classification is cardio exercise, and the other is resistance or weight training, and both of those exercises do two distinct things to the body.

First, described at a basic level cardiovascular exercise is going to strengthen the cardiovascular system. It's any exercise that raises your heart rate to at least 50% of it's maximum level. By doing cardiovascular exercise we strengthen our bodies ability to deliver oxygen to the cells in our muscles, and we strengthen our heart, which is a muscle as well.

Weight training or resistance training builds the musculoskeletal system — the skeleton and skeletal muscle. Resistance training is an exercise that causes skeletal muscle to contract against external resistance. Consistent weight training leads to increases in strength, tone, mass, and/or endurance. Basically it makes muscles bigger and stronger.

But in no way and in no clinical study, meaning no study where they actually performed an experiment, have they ever been able to prove that exercise alone causes fat loss. It doesn't. It causes strength building, whether that's strength building of the cardiovascular system or the musculoskeletal system.

For example, if we go back in time to maybe the '40s or the '50s, or a time when we heard our parents say that they had to "work up an appetite," well.. how would they do that? One of the ways that we would work up an appetite was we would put in a long, hard day of work, of physical work, and it would increase our hunger.

So one way that exercise can actually make us fat is that we'll want to eat more calories as a result of doing more physical exertion. Usually if we are not used to tracking the amount of exercise we do we'll also great overestimate the calories we burned, and we underestimate the calories we eat afterward. If we don't understand that sugar and refined carbohydrates increase our fat storage hormone we'll also think that we can "indulge tonight and burn it off tomorrow." But you can't out exercise bad eating.

Another issue for many people, especially people who have been chronically overweight, or people who are experiencing a lot of pain throughout the body, or if they have symptoms of heart disease, is that they're having a systemic (ie: throughout the body) over-inflammatory response. Inflammation can be classified as "good" or "bad". The "good" inflammation is the kind we think of as helping us heal from a wound or sickness (think about a fever when we catch a cold or the flu. The fever is inflammation killing off virus or bacteria.) But "bad" inflammation is the kind linked to heart disease or Type 2 Diabetes and it's this type of inflammation that can make exercise work against you.

Fat cells are capable of creating chemical signals that lead to chronic inflammation. But they mainly do so when you habitually eat too many calories and sugar. These chemical signals also mess with the way that insulin works in our bodies, aggravating insulin resistance. Remember, insulin is our fat storage hormone. These responses in the body cause weight gain. Now lets say you decide to exercise on top of that, and you increase the inflammation. Therefore, you increase the body's ability to gain weight and decrease its ability to lose weight, which is why many of my clients, before they come in to me, will say something like,

> "I don't understand what's going on. I'm working out, I'm increasing my activity, I'm busting my butt in the gym and my body doesn't look any different. It's not any smaller and it doesn't weigh any less."

If fat cells, among other factors, contribute to chronic inflammation, then it's reasonable to expect that weight gain, especially in the form of fat tissue, also contributes to chronic inflammation. Add an inflammatory process like exercise into the equation without removing or controlling other dietary or hormonal issues and you have a perfect storm, a trifecta of weight gain and fat storage. And as we continue to gain weight, fat cells can expand beyond their capacity of storing our extra calories as fat. When this happens, they turn on and add to the inflammation already present in our bodies. At this point, the body is overloaded from different directions and spiraling downward, and all the while the person is exercising trying to improve their health.

Exercise and Hormones

So let's go back to that example of the hormonal imbalance. If I have a client who's eating a diet that's high in sugar —whether it's a hidden sugar or a known one, right — they're having some kind of carbohydrate-heavy diet that's rich in refined or processed carbohydrate. When they're eating those foods, they're triggering an insulin response. Insulin suppresses glucagon, and we said glucagon burns fat. And insulin makes the body store fat. So here's what that means. That means you might decide that you want to go on a diet, and maybe left the house early, and you didn't have time to bring your food with you, so you thought,

"Well, you know what? I'm on a diet, so I'm just going to lower my calories. I'm going to hit up a coffee place and I'm going to have small coffee. I'm going to put a little bit of whipped cream on it, maybe a couple shots of syrup, but that's all I'm going to have.

"Now, I'm a smart person. I know that that's probably 400 calories, but that's okay because I'm going to go to the gym at lunch and I'm going to bust it up and I'm going to burn 500 calories." And you do, you make good on your promise, right? You go into the gym and you burn 500 calories.

The calories in, calories out model tells us that, "I should've burned or be in a deficit of 100 calories." But because that item that you ate in the morning made your body secrete insulin, and insulin stops your body from burning fat, all you did with those 500 calories is burn sugar during the workout.

Whether that was sugar from food in your stomach, sugar that the body stores as fuel like the glycogen, or when it runs out of those two storage sites, it'll actually start breaking down your skeletal muscle and burning that instead, because muscle breaks down to sugar.

The one fuel it will not go after is the one fuel you're in there trying to burn, which is body fat. Depending on which expert you talk to, weight loss is 80 - 85% nutrition. Exercising without

24

having your diet properly dialed in will lead to frustration, and potential injury.. but not fat loss.

Exercising and Toxicity

Basically, it's the same thing all over again. If the body is in a highly toxic environment, the toxin is being stored in the fat cell, and as a result my body's going to be resistant to burning it.

So when I exercise, again, my body's not going to reach for the fat cell because it doesn't want to release the toxin. It's smart, it doesn't want to make us sick. So it's going to protect any cells that are filled with toxicity.

It'll look for an alternative fuel source, but even more important than that is that if there's too much toxin built up in the liver, any fat that is being released by the body is not being properly broken down and converted, so it just gets reabsorbed again.

So again, if the body can't adequately get into the fat stores, it will have to look for an alternate fuel source, which, again, is either going to be your muscle or any sugar that's cruising through the body.

Chapter Four

What Is A Metabolic Program and Can It Help Me Lose Weight?

Up to now a solid argument has been made that a calories in, calories out <u>only</u> type of approach isn't the best one. While the deficit between how much we burn in calories on a daily basis and how many calories are consumed are critical to losing weight, the second half of this rule with my clients is this:

The type of calorie consumed determines the type of weight you will lose.

Therefore the difference between a metabolic program and a calorie reduction program is: calorie reduction is simply trying to create a calorie deficit in some way, while a metabolic program will identify the specific metabolic dysfunction that is preventing a person from losing weight and keeping it off.

With the calories in / calories out model we start with the premise that there's 3,500 calories in a pound of body fat. Meaning that in order to lose one pound of body fat I have to create a deficit in some way of 3,500 calories. Say through the course of a week I want to lose 2 pounds, and I do that by eating 500 calories less every day that what my body needs and exercising 500 calories for a day. That created a deficit of approximately 7,000 calories and I should potentially burn two pounds. That's the calories in, calories out model.

However, what many people who try to diet find is that while the math might add up, what the body actually does on the scale doesn't reflect that at all and the amount of fat they lose is actually much smaller. In addition they plateau often, they are frequently hungry, usually craving, and the body starts gaining weight back as soon as they stop the diet. This is what I put up with for most of my dieting career until I discovered methods to correct metabolism.

A metabolic program is where you're going to identify what specific parts of the metabolism have been damaged, and correct the dysfunction at the same time as doing a calorie deficit.

When we do the metabolic program combined with a calorie deficit, the math does not add up either, same as it did with the calories in, calories out. But the difference in this scenario is it's *actually accelerated*. It goes above and beyond because when the body starts getting these metabolic dysfunctions corrected, it sheds the symptom of obesity. The body will actually accelerate in its ability to lose weight.

By only concentrating on a calories in / calories out approach to losing weight there are significant disadvantages that set the dieter up for failure. The most important of these is failing to correct the metabolic syndrome. Discussing metabolic syndrome is actually a great thing to do because unfortunately, most people do not know what that is.

The metabolic syndrome clusters at least 3 out of 5 medical conditions and is the precursor to the major lifestyle diseases that are plaguing our country, particularly cardiovascular disease and diabetes. If you have at least 3 of the 5 conditions listed, then you are clinically diagnosed with having Metabolic Syndrome:

- Abdominal or centrally-located obesity (are you shaped like an apple)

- High blood pressure

- High blood sugar or elevated plasma glucose

- High serum triglycerides

- Low levels of high-density lipoprotein (HDL) levels

However, even if you have less than the 5 conditions listed above, the chances that you have a dysfunctioning metabolism are high. So what are the top seven leading causes of death in our country at this time, at the time of the writing of this book?

- Heart disease

- Cancer

- Chronic lower respiratory disease

- Accidents (unintentional injuries)

- Stroke

- Alzheimer's disease

- Diabetes

Out of the seven leading causes of death in our country, 5 of them are end result consequences of metabolic syndrome. Meaning when we trace all of those back to their primary starting point, they all start with something called a "dysfunction" in the metabolism. Certain forms of cancer related to metabolic dysfunction specifically for a man might be prostate cancer, for a woman it might be breast, both might have colorectal cancer or some derivative. In regards to Alzheimer's disease, more and more studies are revealing that insulin resistance is directly related to Alzheimer's, with many researchers citing that type 2 diabetes can potentially serve as a co-factor or co-contributor in the creation of Alzheimer's disease or it's progression[1].

Therefore, by using a metabolic program to reduce body fat, we're going to identify those precursors that are leading the client not only to obesity, but to those five major lifestyle diseases that are plaguing the country, and correct them. Now not only will you be losing weight, losing it at an accelerated pace, doing it without hormonal hunger, and sharp reduction of cravings, but turning around the leading causes of death that are effecting most of the country.

Chapter Five

How Do I Eliminate Compulsive Overeating or Binge Behavior?

Compulsive overeaters, or binge eaters, are people who engage in short feasts wherein they consume a large amount of calories. Because they are different than bulimics in that they do not purge after these episodes, the then do gain weight. Compulsive overeating is often driven by certain triggers or stimuli in the environment or our habits or surroundings that we're not necessarily aware of, that can trigger us to eat too much.

So examples of stimuli could be things such as a stress response: death in the family, loss of a job, relationship stress, physical trauma. It could also be things like a social response: how we're supposed to behave in social situations such as parties, events, or habitual behaviors. When we have these conditions, we will actually seek out an environment that will allow us to compulsively overeat.

This is important because if you're solution up until now is doing the calories in, calories out approach and you're not correcting these metabolic issues, most people will suffer from: abnormally high levels of hunger, they will deal with cravings on a consistent basis, and scale weight plateaus will be common and frequent. This means they will rely on their willpower alone to get them through it, and the problem is willpower always runs out.

And so what happens for most of us is we start seeing cravings showing up, and we'll deny the cravings initially, but eventually the body will win out because what you are struggling with is a biochemical reaction and an addictive response.

And so when you finally give in, not only do you give into the behavior, but you don't give in with a little bit. You give in with an abnormally large amount of food, usually a carbohydrate or sugar-laden one. This binging or compulsive eating on sugar and refined carbohydrates. The reason the compulsive eating and the sugar are tied in is because sugar is an addictive substance.

Sugar has been identified as a chronic — meaning it takes a long time — dose-dependent — so it depends on how much you eat — hepatotoxin and neurotoxin. So it is literally a poison both to the liver and to the brain. So what happens is, these chemical pathways are developed that reinforce the destructive cycle of addiction. The more foods that you eat that have sugar in them or break down into sugar, the more you chemically hijack the brain just as you would if you decided that you were using or abusing tobacco, alcohol, or even worse, a pharmaceutical like cocaine or heroin, it has the exact same response. So suddenly, you are not fighting a behavioral problem, you are fighting an addiction problem.

Techniques to Control Binge Eating

An incredibly effective technique that people have used to control, so for the binging behavior, is something called "EFT" or Emotional Freedom Technique. Emotional Freedom Technique is a form of counseling intervention that draws on various theories of alternative medicine including acupuncture, neuro-linguistic programming, energy medicine, and Thought Field Therapy (TFT).

If you're drawn to compulsive eating or binge behavior that you feel is rooted in emotional or stress response issues, then EFT is simple and effective, and can rapidly help you control your emotional food cravings. Most of us don't understand how destructive the underlying emotional turmoil can be and that emotional well-being is essential to their physical health. In fact, in terms of dieting for weight loss, if these emotional issues — whether small or serious traumas from the past — are suppressed, most people is the who lose weight will often fail at keeping it off.

Maintaining negative thoughts and feelings while trying to take physical steps to improve your body is one of the reasons we see a 95% failure rate, especially in those individuals who, for all intents and purposes, are following other healthy measures to reduce their body fat percentage and reach and maintain their goal weight. Therefore, properly identifying these negative thoughts and feelings and successfully mediating them is absolutely imperative to achieve optimal physical health.

Unfortunately, many people shun this notion, not because it doesn't make sense, but because 1) they don't understand the importance of it or 2) they don't understand how it can be done. In contrast to traditional psychological approaches, EFT has shown to be a far better, not to mention inexpensive, solution. EFT can help you:

Additional benefits to applying EFT technique include:

- Relieving most emotional traumas

- Abolish phobias and post-traumatic stress

- Shatter food cravings that sabotage your health

- Eliminate or significantly reduce most physical pain and discomfort

Let's identify exactly how someone can start using this

technique for themselves. Basically, what Emotional Freedom Technique is, is applying repeated taps to different areas of the body to interfere with nervous system impulses to the brain. This tapping pattern briefly interrupts the connection in the nervous system to the brain that's driving the behavior.

The EFT Basic Tapping Technique has only 5 brief steps and takes very little effort to learn. Once memorized, each round of it can be performed in about 30 seconds. It will take some practice, of course, but after a few tries the whole process becomes familiar and you can do it in your sleep. You will then have a permanent tool that you can use for a lifetime. During the session use focused wording that tunes you into the negative issue that you would like to diminish. This wording is an essential part of the process because it tells our system what we are working on. Negative emotions come about because we are tuned into certain thoughts or circumstances which, in turn, cause our energy systems to disrupt.

The Five Step Basic EFT Technique

Step 1: Identify the Negative Issue or Behavior

This could be a bad habit with eating, a craving when first removing an unwanted or unhealthy food from the diet, or dealing with an unexpected exposure to a binge related food.

Step 2: Identify The Initial Intensity of the Negative Response

Here you establish a before level of the issue's intensity by assigning a number to it on a 0-10 scale where 10 is the worst the issue has ever been and 0 is no problem whatsoever. This serves as a benchmark so we can compare our progress after each round of The EFT Technique.

Step 3: Design a Tapping Phrase

There are two steps to designing a tapping phrase. The first half of the phrase identifies or acknowledges the negative behavior. In the 2nd half of the phrase you accept yourself in spite of the negative behavior. Some examples of Tapping Phrases include:

> *"Even though I can't stop drinking soda, I deeply and completely accept myself."*

> *"Even though I can't seem to stop eating sugar, I completely love and accept myself."*

Step 4: Perform the Sequence

This is the workhorse part of The EFT Technique that stimulates/ interrupts the neural impulses between the body and the brain. To perform it, you tap each of the points shown in the Sequence Points listed while saying the Reminder Phrase that you designed in the previous step. The sequence of tapping points always follow the same sequence order and are as follows:

The Karate Chop Point

The Karate Chop point (abbreviated KC) is located at the center of the fleshy part of the outside of your hand (either hand) between the top of the wrist and the base of the baby finger or....stated differently....the part of your hand you would use to deliver a karate chop. Note: It is during this point that your main tapping phrase that you created in step 3 is stated. Therefore, spend about 15 seconds here re-stating the phrase before moving on.

Medial (or inner) Eyebrow

Where the hairline of the eyebrow begins closest to the nose.

Temple

On the side of the face at eye level, on the same side as the previous point.

Under Inner Eye

On the bone under an eye about 1 inch below your pupil.

Under Nose

On the small area between the bottom of your nose and the top of your upper lip.

Under Mouth

Midway between the point of your chin and the bottom of your lower lip. It is not directly on the point of the chin, but just above it.

Inner Collarbone

The junction where the sternum (breastbone), collarbone and the first rib meet.

Under Arm

On the side of the body, at a point even with the nipple (for men) or in the middle of the bra strap (for women). It is about 4 inches below the armpit.

While performing the remaining points of the tapping sequence, the tapping phrase is quite simple as you need only identify the issue with some brief wording. Depending on your issue, you might say the following at each tapping point....

"Can't stop eating sugar"

"This soda pop craving"

"This difficulty losing weight"

Step 5: Test the Intensity Again

Finally, you establish an "after" level of the issue's intensity by assigning a number to it on a 0-10 scale. You compare this with the before level to see how much progress you have made. If you are not down to zero then repeat the process until you either achieve zero or plateau at some level. Usually, just one cycle, which takes 30 seconds or less, can drop a craving or a negative behavior by a minimum of 50 percent and could be done in under 60 seconds.

Alternative Approach to Stopping Binge Behavior

Many times when people struggle with binge behavior or compulsive eating, they might do therapy sessions to try to identify, "Are there hidden triggers? Was I in an abusive relationship? Am I being heavy to try to protect myself from something? Am I depressed? Am I showing clinical, mental deficiencies?" But for a great majority of the public, they don't have these hidden issues that might be driving a compulsive behavior or a binge behavior.

This was the case for me. There was no emotional or physical trauma that I could identify, I just simply liked to eat food. When I started treating clients I found that many of them were the same way. What I was able to help them recognize is that what had developed was basically a neural pathway that started with having a craving and consistently reacting to it with the unwanted behavior. As a result, the behavior was reinforced. So the brain gave you an impulse, but it couldn't voluntarily control your motion. But because you respond to the impulse, and because it's usually associated (in this case) with eating a hyperstimuating or addictive food, you were "positively rewarded" and this encouraged the brain to reinforce and repeat the impulse.

For example: Let's say there's a cupcake sitting on the kitchen counter. And it's 9:00 at night and it's sitting right there. Even though your brain might give you the urge and tell you, "I want to have that. I want to eat that cupcake," it cannot physically make you put your hand out, grab the cupcake and eat it. That is a voluntary response. You have to voluntarily do it.

So a very effective way of eliminating binge behavior, compulsive behavior, is basically, while hearing the impulse and recognizing that it's there, *you don't act on it.*

So an example of that might be: back in the day before answering machines and voice mail, if the phone rang in our house, but there was nothing there to answer it .... if you were sitting there, it was very difficult not to go over and answer the phone. We were just hardwired that if the phone's ringing, we have to answer the phone.

What this technique is basically saying what you want to do is, instead of going over there and fighting the urge to answer the phone or reaching over and doing it, you recognize that the phone is ringing, but you continue with whatever activity that you're currently doing. You don't feed it, you don't fight it, you just recognize, "Yes, I hear you," and keep doing the original behavior that you're doing. What happens is, every time that you're able to recognize the impulse but not act on it, you weaken the neural pathway that's sending the impulse. Because the brain is dynamic, or it's plastic (meaning that it changes), what it will actually do is dissolve that neural pathway, and then you won't have that compulsive reaction anymore. You won't have the reaction, because you stop feeding and rewarding it.

In the phone example it means if someone keeps calling (the nerve impulse) but you just sit there and don't answer the phone, eventually not only will the phone stop ringing at that instance but if you keep avoiding answering the phone the person on the other end will just stop calling altogether. They've learned that they can not contact you that way.

Chapter Six

How Can I Achieve Long-Term Success for Weight Loss?

What many people don't know is that the dieting process or losing weight is a two-fold process. The first process is going from your original weight to your target weight. First of all, getting to the target weight might be hard enough, but when we get there, what the majority of us will do is we'll say, "Woohoo, I'm at goal! I'm done! Bring on the pie, bring on the party! I've completed my job." No, you haven't. What you've completed is **step one**. Step two is you have to maintain that weight and you have to maintain it for a minimum of 12 to 18 months before you have retrained that hypothalamus that this is the new goal weight.

To determine target weight most people will pick a certain number that felt right to them or a number in their past, or they'll pick a clothing size. As long as it's an achievable number, and most numbers are achievable, it can be done. Where the diet programs often fail us is not teaching us that by dieting for any length of time we have to some effect slowed down the rate that our body burns calories. This means that once we achieve our target weight some kind of reverse dieting process is necessary to maximize the number of calories we can eat again without regaining the weight we lost.

So what is reverse dieting? Well again, when you diet for any length of time, you will slow down the amount of calories your body burns every day. So if you decided to do a 1,300-calorie diet and you get to your goal weight doing that, and then the very next day you decide, "I'm done with my goal and I'm going to go back to a 2,000-calorie diet," technically you're going to have a 700 calorie-a-day surplus. Jumping your calories up to back up to original levels in short order often results in quickly gaining back the weight you've lost. What reverse dieting accomplishes is slowly increasing the calories while monitoring the scale to let the body slowly increase its metabolism back to the max amount of calories you want to eat in a day.

Besides just monitoring the number of calories eating during a day and reversing it to it's maximum, another crucial concept of reverse dieting is food balancing. This means understanding what your specific macronutrient content should be based on your family history, activity levels, and body composition goals. The simple definition of a macronutrient is basically, protein, carbohydrates and fat. And the body looks and feels differently depending on how those numbers are constructed in not only our weight loss diet, but our maintenance diet as well.

For example, many physique competitors during "contest prep" (the diet followed before a stage competition) are looking to maximize muscle gain while having a low to very low percentage of body fat. As a result they might manipulate their protein intake to roughly half a gram to a gram per pound of body weight. If somebody weighs 170 pounds and they're a male, they're probably going to want to have 170 grams of protein a day. If they're female, they might drop it down to 140 or 130, and that amount of protein on a daily basis will help keep you full, will help keep you satiated, and will help protect muscle while weight training and applying cardio exercise in the weeks preparing for the competition.

How Can I Travel and Keep Weight Off?

For many people staying on track, losing weight, and keeping it off can be fraught with several difficulties. This is especially true in the United States where it is well documented that we are the fattest nation on the planet. A common obstacle I hear from my clients goes something like this, "Well, my problem is I travel a lot or I entertain a lot, and I'm not able to keep my goal weight long-term because of these conditions."

By using a method called IIFYM, which stands for If It Fits Your Macros — you can calculate your average daily expenditure and break down the macronutrient amounts to fit your body composition goals. Once this is accomplished these numbers can be plugged into any number of free calorie tracking apps. Tracking these macro numbers; keeping a loose eye on them on a daily basis can literally let you go anywhere and eat anything, as long as it fits within the numbers you selected. It also allows you to keep the weight off, and keep it off long-term. For all of my weight loss clients, I design not only the phase where they are focused on reducing body fat and correcting metabolism, but also two additional phases where the metabolism is tested to make sure it's resistant, as well as this final maintenance phase. All three phases are critical for long term weight loss success.

Food Preparation in Long-Term Success

There's an old adage that goes something like this, "If you fail to plan, you're planning to fail," and nowhere else that I know of is it more critical than with weight loss and public health as it is for any other industry, at least in this country. If fat loss, or just your overall health for that matter, is of any importance to you it's imperative that you create some kind of battle plan to fight for it. If you do not, you will become a statistic and fall victim to Metabolic Syndrome and all it's ugly consequences. Because of this, I teach my clients the importance of food preparation or "food prep" for short. When I first bring up the idea of food preparation, many of my clients feel overwhelmed or that it's too out of reach, but that's simply because it's not a habit.. yet. But the more you work at it, the better you become. And it's an essential part of weight loss. All my most successful clients incorporated meal planning and preparation as part of their weight loss journey.

So to start, what is food prep? Food prep simply put is buying, preparing and storing your food ahead of time so that it's ready for you when you need it. It's usually done on a weekly basis, but doesn't have to be because for many that can be pretty overwhelming in the beginning. My recommendation is to start slow. The first week or two prep for two to three days at a time with simple recipes and as you get comfortable with the process you can prepare more.

So for my metabolic program it might look something like this:

I'm going to buy a weeks' worth of groceries that's in my program. I'm going to go home, I'm going to prepare it all and I'm going to portion it out for the week, because as all of us know, we're all busy, we're all stressed and we all have things that show up unexpectedly.

So in the Starbucks example that I used in a previous chapter, if I decided Sunday night I want to start a diet, but Monday I woke up late or something happened and I just had to run out the door, without my food prep habit I'm susceptible to the environment. If you allow yourself to be susceptible to your environment, you will always — especially in America — be a victim to the environment and you will fail at that diet. So you really have to take the steps to plan.

Stick with healthy recipes you already know. Depending on the recipe or food item, you can make enough to store in the refrigerator, the freezer, or both. The foods you prep also does not all have to be cooked. They could be cut up fruits or vegetables, healthy grains, etc.. but a critical step is splitting the food into meals ahead of time. In the beginning, choose the recipes that if made ahead of time, would make the biggest difference in getting you to your goals. In other words, prioritize your meals. And remember that even the smallest amount of food prep makes a difference. This way if an emergency or an unusual circumstance comes up, you're prepared for it.

Chapter Seven

How Do I Do This On My Own?

I tell every client, "There's going to be four things that will determine whether or not you will lose weight and keep it off. One is hunger, one is cravings, one is habit, and one is surroundings." Let's get into them one by one.

The first factor is hunger. To keep it simplified for the scope of this book there are basically two types of hunger we will talk about here. There's physical hunger, where your body is physically in need of food, and then there's hormonal hunger, which is hunger driven by hormones. When I first start working with a client, my job is to evaluate if there's any metabolic dysfunction. Factors such as toxicity, acidity, inflammation, medications etc. can trigger hormonal hunger. Also, if my client has been eating the Standard American Diet then quite often their insulin levels have been too high. This causes not only the creation and storage of body fat, but that also means they're craving sugar; all driven by an insulin imbalance.

When we start correcting those issues and converting the body from burning sugar to burning fat, the body's used to getting a certain kind of fuel. As a result it doesn't have the hormones in place to burn body fat efficiently, so it thinks it's hungry even though it's getting calories and nourishment. That's an example of hormonal hunger. When insulin is high, our hunger responses are always very, very fast because as the body gets rid of the blood sugar, the hormone of insulin demands more.

The second factor that will determine how successful someone will be at losing weight is cravings. Cravings can sabotage weight loss. A big part of this comes from two deficits in our diet: nutritional deficiency and the continuous eating of acidic and inflammatory foods. These two problems are compounded as we eat American foods on a daily basis and lower the body's pH. There are two types of pH values for humans. One is blood pH and the second is the pH of the digestive tract. When I discuss pH with my client I'm referring to their digestive tract pH, which can have varied ranges depending on which part of the digestive tract is being discussed. If the body is struggling with a health problem, there is a high likelihood that you are acidic. In fact, in 1922 there was a scientist named Otto Warburg, who determined that if the body's pH stayed slightly alkaline, your body physically can't produce cancer cells.

But there are several things that can make our body acidic. One is an acid forming diet, such as the bottled water we drink and a heavily processed diet, filled with sugar and refined carbohydrates. Another is pharmaceuticals, because pharmaceuticals are built off of an acid base, so as you keep taking your daily dose of medication, your pH goes lower.

A nasty side effect of an acidic pH is that as the pH goes down, the body craves pH foods. People in our country are led to believe that what they're dealing with is a behavioral problem or an inability to have enough willpower when they fall off their diet. Actually it is a chemical reaction to their pH environment, to their toxic environment. And so what we find is if we eliminate that toxicity and raise the pH back up, the cravings problem goes away. They actually don't have the craving for the food, so it's much easier to stay on a program long-term if you're not suffering from hunger and cravings in the first place.

Next is converting your habits, because they'll make or break you. Every habit that you have is technically a neural pathway that you've created as a response to neural impulses. Most times when we do a program on our own, we have a really hard time controlling the reaction to that neural impulse, even if we know that our response to it is a voluntary one. The impulse can't make us buy our Friday night pizza, but because the impulse was reinforced for a particularly long period of time, many people feel helpless to resist.

Most people when they embark on a new weight loss program they are battling all four of these elements — hunger, cravings, habit and surroundings. By using a customized metabolic program that's specifically design for the individual, the hunger and cravings issue is minimized or removed altogether. Now it becomes much easier to break that neural reaction that we have as a result of our habits.

Finally we have to learn how to navigate our surroundings. This is important because we live on the fattest country on the planet. Eighty percent of our population is classified as overweight. Twenty-nine percent of us are now classified as obese, meaning that we have a BMI of 29 or higher. And it's not getting any better, and we'll probably not get better in our lifetime. If you don't learn where these metabolically damaging foods are, or if you believe what you're being told is healthy when it's really not, you will never be able to keep the weight off long-term, which is the biggest reason we have a 95 percent failure rate in our country. And 95 percent of all people who lose weight will gain it back within a year, meaning that only one in 20 can keep it off for more than 12 months, and only one in 50 can keep it off for five years. If you don't learn where it's hiding, you're never going to reach that five percent.

Epilogue

So what have we covered in the course of this book…?

Firstly, let me say at the outset that never during the entire course of my weight loss problem did I ever think that it was a blessing. It was a burden, it was shameful, and it was always something I felt I couldn't overcome. What a difference a few short years makes.

In my personal weight loss journey I discovered so many things I didn't know. I graduated from college with a Human Biology degree and from chiropractic college with a doctorate, yet I didn't know about these basic metabolic factors and what a huge impact they had on my ability to lose weight and keep it off. And even if I had some of the knowledge, I had no clue how to apply it to me.

I believed the grocery stores, the restaurants, and the so-called "healthy products" when they told me that by cutting the calories and removing the fat they would help me with my weight problem. I believed that because licorice was "fat free" it was okay for me to eat it. What I now know is they lied and fed me misinformation. As I switched out my dressings for lower fat versions, my regular soda for diet, and my white pasta with whole wheat, I thought I was doing my body a favor. Since the age of 19 I beat myself up in the gym. Going on the premise that a calorie is a calorie I was constantly trying to make up for over eating by over exercising. While I could do cardio machines like a pro, I mistakenly avoided the weight section because I thought they would only make me bigger. What a difference a few short years makes.

Now I know that not all calories are created equal and that, in fact, many times I could be damaging the body with exercise simply because I was burning the wrong type of fuel during the activity. I wanted to be burning body fat, but all I was burning was sugar. And by avoiding the weight room I only escalated the problem by incinerating my muscle to fuel me through the workouts when the stored sugar ran out.

But I was fortunate. In 2009 I found that there was a different way. A better way. I found a way to apply a metabolic program to my weight loss problem and discovered that I could lose weight: at a more accelerated rate than ever before, without hunger, without cravings, and with less exercise than I had previously done on any program. *But that was only half my reward.* Even if all those issues were still in place the real reward was when I stopped doing my program... *and the weight stayed off.* Never in my life had I experienced that before.

In the seven years since I completed my personal metabolic program I learned what was causing my compulsive eating and binge behavior. And I learned how to control it until it was corrected. I learned what I needed to have in place to create long term, successful weight loss not only for myself, but for hundreds of clients in the three years since I offered my metabolic program to the public.

And, ultimately, I was able to discover what I felt was the most important part of this entire formula: *the ability to achieve long-term, successful weight loss.* The sad truth of it is we live in a country where 95% of people who lose weight gain it back within one year. Only 1 person in 50 who lose weight keep it off for over 5 years. I have beaten both of those odds, which puts me in an ultra elite category when it comes to weight loss. I am not saying this to brag to you. I'm saying it because I have since then learned how to duplicate those results in my clients. As a result, many of my clients get their confidence back, they look better, they feel better, get off their medications, and go on to lead healthier, more productive lives. Do they all experience this? No, because if someone isn't ready to make a change, *no program can help them. None. Period.*

Ultimately only you can decide if you're ready to make a change. Only you can decide if you're tired of being mislead by the numerous powers-that-be when talking about the public health sector: the medical community, the pharmaceutical community, the food manufacturers, and even the diet and fitness industry. And only you can decide if you're ready to take the information provided in this book and build off it, use it as a springboard to advance your knowledge, regain your health and vitality, and let's say it… look as good as you want to look, no matter what obstacle you may be facing.

If you don't feel this is a task you can face alone, I am always here to help. What I would like to do is personally help you get the results you desire so I've put together a very special no cost, no obligation, very limited time offer for you.

$47.00 5 Step TOTAL

Metabolic Weight Loss Evaluation…

For Only $19.00

I will set time aside to personally meet with you and lay out a customized plan so you can reach your goal weight and stay there.

During Our Time Together You Will Discover

- _Your_ key metabolic issues that are preventing you from losing weight

- Why the diets you've tried in the past haven't worked and how to correct it

- What type of exercise (if any) will help you reach your goals fast

- The Top 10 Habits Of Long-Term Successful Dieters

- FOUR Steps To Beat Food Addiction, Plus 10 Facts That Might Just Shock You

I'm so confident that you'll find the "5 Step TOTAL Metabolic Weight Loss Evaluation" valuable that I'm going to give you a ...

100% Risk Free Guarantee

Although your consultation is only $19.00, I do know that your time is valuable. I also understand you might be wondering if it's as valuable as I say it is so I am putting my money where my mouth is. If, after our time together, you don't feel it was worth your time, just tell me and I will give you double your money back.

Imagine if you could wave a magic wand and look better, feel better by reaching your goal weight and staying there.

I can help you make that happen. The first step it's call my office at 866–515–0101, ask to speak to Pat and tell her, "I want to take advantage of Dr. Nash's 5 Step TOTAL Metabolic Weight Loss Evaluation." And she will get you all set up.

Please don't wait to call. I only have limited spaces to do these reduced fee consultations and I'd hate for you to get all the way to the end of this book and not get one of them.

There is no cost or obligation. Call Pat right now while it's still fresh on your mind.

Wishing You Ultimate Health & Happiness,

Dr. Kathleen Nash, D.C.

P.S. I understand if you're a bit skeptical. Many of my happy clients felt the same way before they met with me but if you visit my website at www.drnash.com you can discover for yourself what kind of results they found.

Bonus Chapter

The SIX Factors That Will Ultimately Determine Rate Of Weight Loss

In my own experience, and in watching hundreds of clients go through their own personal transformations, there are SIX things that will ultimately determine rate of weight loss:

Number of Calories

Finding the right range of calories for an individual to lose weight is a personalized and subjective procedure. In my office, I determine this for my clients but in a book there is no easy answer. However, there are some good formulas that can give someone a head start.

Quality of Calories

The more your diet is comprised of real whole unprocessed food, the faster your body will lose weight. Foods that contain: sugar, refined carbohydrates, chemicals and additives, and processing methods usually interfere with the body's ability to lose body fat which is the main goal. A person may lose weight and be rewarded on the scale in the short term, but it is usually a mixture of body fat, water, and lean mass (muscle, organ, and bone density) that is lost. As a result of less body fat lost per pound, people who incorporate more processed foods into their diet program will either have to supplement with some form of physical training or be satisfied with a less than ideal looking physique.

Supplementation for Metabolic Correction

After quality and quantity of calories is what I call "maxed", meaning there's very little left to change, supplementation can be considered to boost your weight loss efforts. In my office, I use physician grade supplementation but only after I've identified in an evaluation what my client's metabolic dysfunctions are. Having someone take a supplement for a condition they don't have is basically just having them pour money down the toilet… literally. Before you consider using any form supplementation in your personal weight loss efforts, I highly recommend maximizing the other items I've listed here or hiring a metabolic specialist to determine what specific supplementation you would need to fit your lifestyle and physique goals.

Water Intake

Daily water intake is an integral part of any weight loss program. From it's toxin eliminating effects to it's muscle rehydration it's an important part to max out on a daily basis. Researchers in Germany even report that water consumption increases the rate at which people burn calories. Spacing out your water consumption throughout the day will ensure that your body is replenished and gets rid of excess water weight. If you only consume water when you are thirsty then your body will be depleted of necessary fluids and retain the water weight. A good rule of thumb of how much water you need is based on the color of your urine. If you have a dark yellow-colored urine it is a strong indication that you need more fluids in your body. For healthy, light-colored urine, it is important to drink a glass of water when you wake up in the morning and then every two hours. Even after you use the restroom, drink another glass of water so that your body is plenty replenished.

Activity Level

This means exercise. Only you can decide how much you want to max that out. You can either:

1. Increase the frequency that you exercise. How many days a week do you currently add regular exercise to your routine? If it is 6 to 7 days a week you are maxed.

2. Increase the duration that you exercise. 1 to 2 hours a day is the maximum we would recommend anybody do, and for no longer than a 30 day period at a time. The type of exercise that you choose is entirely up to you and is determined by what your specific physique goals are.

3. Increase the intensity that you exercise. Activity that is easy to do... is easy to do! And will have little to no effect on your rate of weight loss. Therefore, you must work harder to get more out of the exercise. The closer you get to your goal the harder you're going to have to work. It's a law of physics. This could mean lifting heavier weight, adding a new types of activity, incorporating HIIT training, adding extra cardio sessions... the list is endless, and again is a personal and subjective choice which varies from person to person.

Time and Patience

Once you've maxed out the top five things I just outlined, the only thing you can do is <u>keep them going until you reach your goal.</u> Of the six things that I outlined, <u>my program maximizes four of them for you.</u> Because no doctor, weight loss program, or bariatric surgical procedure can control things such as: your family history, your genetic makeup, current medications that can slow your progress, environmental impact on your metabolism up until now, level of compliance, level of activity that you do, and ability to give yourself the time you need to get to your goal, they are left out of mine and every other weight loss program or procedure, because only the patient can have an impact on them. If you have maxed out everything possible in the five things that I outlined, then the only thing you have left is to simply keep them maxed until you reach your goal. There is no way around that.

REFERENCE

1. J Diabetes Sci Technol. 2008 Nov; 2(6): 1101–1113. Published online 2008 Nov.

Made in the USA
Columbia, SC
29 August 2020